MW00768024

Best Copycat Cookbook 2021

The newest and best cookbook for cooking like in top brand restaurants....

Enjoy the tastiest recipes and start cooking as if you were the chef of Panera, Starbucks, Red Lobster and many other restaurants.

Jaqueline Weber

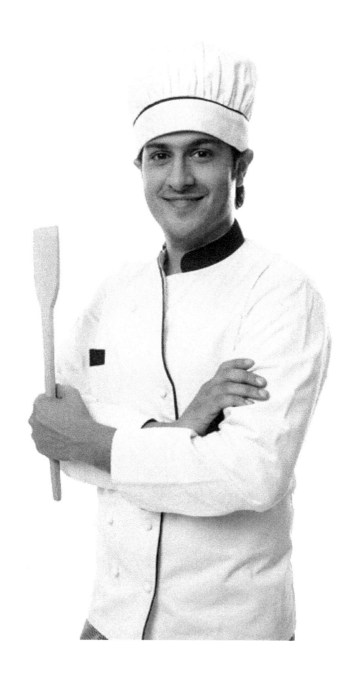

TABLE OF CONTENTS

—

INTRODUCTION

Dining out is one of the things we enjoy the most. The great thing about eating out that makes it more amusing is having a lot of time catching up with friends, a fast drive-through, going out on a hot date, or celebrating a family occasion revolves around food. You may never think you can reconstruct the food you order at Pei Wei, Panda Express, or PF Chang's.

What if you could create traditional restaurant food from the comfort of your home! Exciting, right? You do not leave the house, do not wait in line, and do not waste money on luxurious food — just the mouth-watering taste of your favorite restaurant meals and the guarantee that you can recreate them in your kitchen whenever you want.

Come to think of the money you can save and waiting in line all the time lost. You can make mouth-watering meals without leaving your home, and you'll know more about the ingredients that are being used. Using the simple copycat recipes from the most famous restaurants, you can create your favorite restaurant dishes at home!

Very soon, right before your eyes, you can now start cooking like a high-end restaurant chef and save most of your time! The most significant part about those recipes inclined from the restaurant is that you can twist some ingredients that suit your tastes. The copycat recipe may include grilling meat, but instead, you can always cook it in a skillet or bake it in the oven. Want seafood over poultry or meat, turn with the ingredient you want. Don't like any vegetables or the spiciness level? Only change the right ingredients, and you and your family will be delighted with the meal.

What prompted me to look for those so-called 'secret recipes' is that once I located the one for my favorite well-known dish, I could revel in it every time I desired proper at home.

I also wanted to locate some eating place copycat recipes because you can save numerous cash cooking those dishes yourself. Plus, getting to decide on my portion's length is excellent. I could eat the entire Fonduta myself if I had the chance.

These copycat recipes are tested repeatedly to make sure that you are creating authentic dishes from the restaurant. Expert cooks spend hours tweaking those recipes to get the taste just right. These recipes are as near the real thing as sitting your favorite restaurant proper in your kitchen.

If you have an own family and like to go out to restaurants, but do not enjoy the nasty charge tag related to a terrific meal, then those eating place copycat recipes are for you.

You shouldn't be a trained chef to prepare dinner your pleasant personal meals at home with restaurant copycat recipes. All you need are eating place copycat recipes, the components listed, and get admission to your kitchen.

Visualize impressing your buddies and own family with food that they have most effectively enjoyed at some restaurants, proper from your very own domestic comfort. Visualize how fulfilling it would be to show them that you created those masterpieces within your kitchen's comfort with restaurant copycat recipes!

BREAKFAST

Peach Pancakes

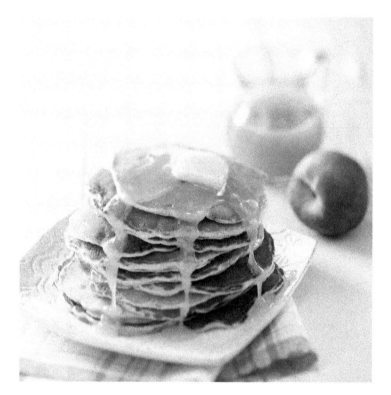

Preparation Time: 10 Minutes

Cooking Time: 10 Minutes

Servings: 6

Ingredients:

- 1 cup whole-wheat flour
- 1 egg, beaten

- 1 teaspoon vanilla extract
- 2 peaches, chopped
- 1 tablespoon margarine
- ½ teaspoon baking powder
- 1 teaspoon apple cider vinegar
- ¼ cup skim milk

Directions:

1. Make the pancake batter: in the mixing bowl mix up eggs, whole-wheat flour, vanilla extract, baking powder, apple cider vinegar, and skim milk.
2. Then melt the margarine in the skillet.
3. Pour the prepared batter in the skillet with the help of the ladle and flatten in the shape of the pancake.
4. Cook the pancakes for 2 minutes from each side over the medium-low heat.
5. Top the cooked pancakes with peaches.

Nutrition: 129 calories, 3.9g protein, 21.5g carbohydrates, 3g fat, 1.3g fiber, 27mg cholesterol, 39mg sodium, 188mg potassium

Breakfast Splits

Preparation Time: 15 Minutes

Cooking Time: 0 Minutes

Servings: 2

Ingredients:

- 2 bananas, peeled
- 4 tablespoons granola
- 2 tablespoons low-fat yogurt
- ½ teaspoon ground cinnamon
- 1 strawberry, chopped

Directions:

1. In the mixing bowl, mix up yogurt with ground cinnamon, and strawberries.
2. Then make the lengthwise cuts in bananas and fill with the yogurt mass.
3. Top the fruits with granola.

Nutrition: 154 calories, 6.8g protein, 45.2g carbohydrates, 8g fat, 6.3g fiber, 1mg cholesterol, 20mg sodium, 635mg potassium

Banana Pancakes

Preparation Time: 10 Minutes

Cooking Time: 15 Minutes

Servings: 5

Ingredients:

- 2 bananas, mashed
- ½ cup 1% milk
- 1 ½ cup whole-grain flour
- 1 teaspoon liquid honey
- 1 teaspoon vanilla extract
- 1 teaspoon baking powder
- 1 tablespoon lemon juice
- 1 tablespoon olive oil

Directions:

1. Mix up mashed bananas and milk.
2. Then add flour, liquid honey, vanilla extract, baking powder, and lemon juice.
3. Whisk the mixture until you get a smooth batter.
4. After this, heat up olive oil in the skillet.
5. When the oil is hot, pour the pancake mixture in the skillet and flatten in the shape of pancakes.

6. Cook them for 1 minute and then flip on another side. Cook the pancakes for 1 minute more.

Nutrition: 207 calories, 6.3g protein, 39.9g carbohydrates, 3.9g fat, 5.7g fiber, 1mg cholesterol, 15mg sodium, 458mg potassium.

Aromatic Breakfast Granola

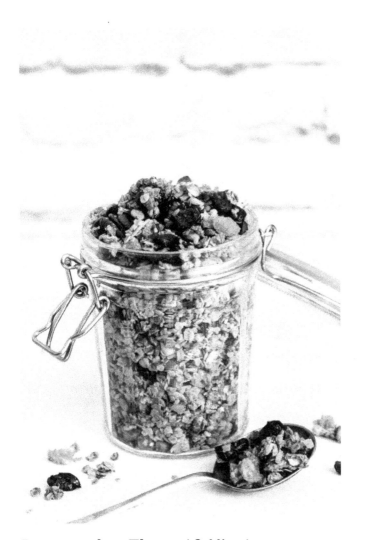

Preparation Time: 10 Minutes

Cooking Time: 25 Minutes

Servings: 2

Ingredients:

- 2 tablespoons avocado oil

- 1 tablespoon liquid honey
- ¼ teaspoon ground cinnamon
- ¼ cup almonds, chopped
- 1 tablespoon chia seeds
- 1 teaspoon sesame seeds
- 2 tablespoons cut oats
- Cooking spray

Directions:

1. Heat up avocado oil and liquid honey until you get a homogenous mixture.
2. Then add ground cinnamon, almonds, chia seeds, sesame seeds, and cut oats.
3. Stir until homogenous.
4. Spray the baking tray with cooking spray and place the almond mixture inside.
5. Flatten it in the shape of a square.
6. Bake the granola at 345F for 20 minutes.
7. Cut it into servings.

Nutrition: 203 calories, 5.7g protein, 22.3g carbohydrates, 11.4g fat, 5.9g fiber, 0mg cholesterol, 2mg sodium, 211mg potassium

Morning Sweet Potatoes

Preparation Time: 5 Minutes

Cooking Time: 20 Minutes

Servings: 2

Ingredients:

- 2 sweet potatoes
- 1 tablespoon chives, chopped
- 2 teaspoons margarine
- ¼ teaspoon chili flakes

Directions:

1. Preheat the oven to 400F.
2. Put the sweet potatoes in the oven and cook them for 20 minutes or until the vegetables are soft.
3. Then cut the sweet potato into halves and top with margarine, chives, and chili flakes. Wait till margarine starts to melt.

Nutrition: 35 calories, 0.1g protein, 0.4g carbohydrates, 3.8g fat, 0.1g fiber, 0mg cholesterol, 45mg sodium, 15mg potassium.

Egg Toasts

Preparation Time: 5 Minutes

Cooking Time: 5 Minutes

Servings: 3

Ingredients:

- 3 eggs
- 3 whole-grain bread slices
- 1 teaspoon olive oil
- ¼ teaspoon minced garlic
- ¼ teaspoon ground black pepper

Directions:

1. Heat up olive oil in the skillet.
2. Crack the eggs inside and cook them for 4 minutes.
3. Meanwhile, rub the bread slices with minced garlic.
4. Top the bread with cooked eggs and sprinkle with ground black pepper.

Nutrition: 157 calories, 8.6g protein, 13.5g carbohydrates, 7.4g fat, 2.1g fiber, 164mg cholesterol, 182mg sodium, 62mg potassium

Sweet Yogurt with Figs

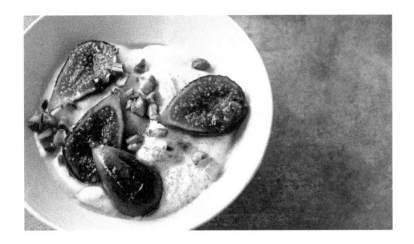

Preparation Time: 5 Minutes

Cooking Time: 0 Minutes

Servings: 1

Ingredients:

- 1/3 cup low-fat yogurt
- 1 teaspoon almond flakes
- 1 fresh fig, chopped
- 1 teaspoon liquid honey
- ¼ teaspoon sesame seeds

Directions:

1. Mix up yogurt and honey and pour the mixture in the serving glass.

2. Top it with chopped fig, almond flakes, and sesame seeds.

Nutrition: 178 calories, 6.2g protein, 24.4g carbohydrates, 6.8g fat, 3.1g fiber, 5mg cholesterol, 44mg sodium, 283mg potassium

Vanilla Toasts

Preparation Time: 10 Minutes

Cooking Time: 5 Minutes

Servings: 3

Ingredients:

- 3 whole-grain bread slices
- 1 teaspoon vanilla extract
- 1 egg, beaten
- 2 tablespoons low-fat sour cream
- 1 tablespoon margarine

Directions:

1. Melt the butter in the skillet.
2. Meanwhile, in the bowl mix up vanilla extract, eggs, and low-fat sour cream.
3. Dip the bread slices in the egg mixture well.
4. Then transfer them in the melted margarine and roast for 2 minutes from each side.

Nutrition: 166 calories, 5.1g protein, 18.7g carbohydrates, 7.9g fat, 2g fiber, 58mg cholesterol, 229mg sodium, 39mg potassium

Raspberry Yogurt

Preparation Time: 5 Minutes

Cooking Time: 0 Minutes

Servings: 2

Ingredients:

- ½ cup low-fat yogurt
- ½ cup raspberries
- 1 teaspoon almond flakes

Directions:

1. Mix up yogurt and raspberries and transfer them in the serving glasses.
2. Top yogurt with almond flakes.

Nutrition: 77 calories, 3.9g protein, 8.6g carbohydrates, 3.4g fat, 2.6g fiber, 4mg cholesterol, 32mg sodium, 192mg potassium

Salsa Eggs

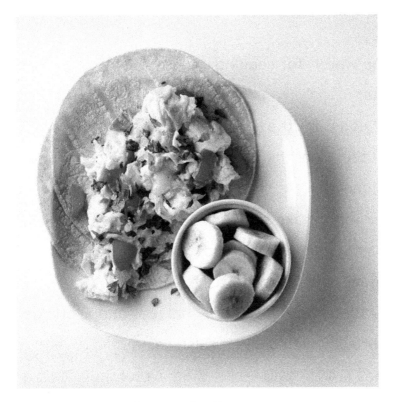

Preparation Time: 10 Minutes

Cooking Time: 10 Minutes

Servings: 4

Ingredients:

- 2 tomatoes, chopped
- 1 chili pepper, chopped
- 2 cucumbers, chopped
- 1 red onion, chopped
- 2 tablespoons parsley, chopped

- 1 tablespoon olive oil
- 1 tablespoon lemon juice
- 4 eggs
- 1 cup water, for cooking eggs

Directions:

1. Put eggs in the water and boil them for 7 minutes. Cool the cooked eggs in the cold water and peel.

2. After this, make salsa salad: mix up tomatoes, chili pepper, cucumbers, red onion, parsley, olive oil, and lemon juice.

3. Cut the eggs into the halves and sprinkle generously with cooked salsa salad.

Nutrition: 140 calories, 7.5g protein, 11.1g carbohydrates, 8.3g fat, 2.2g fiber, 164mg cholesterol, 71mg sodium, 484mg potassium

POULTRY RECIPES

Pei Wei's Kung Páo Chicken

Preparation Time: 15 minutes

Cooking Time: 10 minutes

Servings: 4 - 6

Ingredients

Sauce

- 1 teaspoon red chili paste
- 2 tablespoons low-sodium soy sauce
- 1 tablespoon mirin
- 1 teaspoon seasoned rice wine vinegar
- 1 teaspoon sugar
- ¼ cup chicken broth
- 1 teaspoon cornstarch
- 1 teaspoon dark sesame oil

Stir-fry

1. 1½ lb. boneless, skinless chicken breasts
2. 1 egg, whisked

3. ¼ cup cornstarch

4. ¼ cup canola oil

5. ½ cup frozen crinkle-cut carrots

6. 1 cup sugar snap peas

7. ½ cup dry-roasted peanuts

8. 10 dried red chili peppers, if you want a bit more spice you can also add a dash of red pepper flakes

9. 4 green onions, including green parts, sliced

10.   3 cloves garlic, minced

11.   ½ cup water chestnuts, diced

Directions

- Scourge egg in a small shallow dish. Add the cornstarch to another shallow dish.

- Incorporate all the ingredients for the sauce in a small bowl and set aside. Bread the chicken by first dipping in the egg and then coating with cornstarch. Cook oil over medium-high heat in a large skillet or a wok. When hot, add the coated chicken. Cook through and brown on all sides, then remove chicken to a paper-towel-lined plate to drain.

- Add a bit more oil to the same skillet and heat. When hot, add the peas, chestnuts, and carrots. Cook for 1–2 minutes. Pull out vegetables from the skillet and place them on top of the chicken.
- Add a bit more oil to the skillet, if needed, and quickly sauté the peanuts and chili peppers. They only need to cook for a short time. Add them to the plate with the chicken and vegetables when they are done.
- Stir in green onions, and garlic to the skillet and cook just until fragrant, about 1 minute. Return everything else to the skillet, then add the sauce and stir to make sure everything is coated. Cook until the sauce starts to thicken. Serve with rice.

Nutrition: 684 calories 9g fats 34g protein

Pei Wei's Chicken Lo Mein

Preparation Time: 15 minutes

Cooking Time: 30 minutes

Servings: 4

Ingredients

1. 1½ pounds boneless, skinless chicken breast, sliced very thinly

Marinade

2. 1 tablespoon soy sauce
3. 1½ teaspoons cornstarch
4. 2 tablespoons oyster sauce
5. 2 teaspoons soy sauce
6. ¼ cup beef broth
7. 1 tablespoon sugar

Other ingredients

1. 6 ounces linguine, cooked
2. 1 teaspoon sesame oil
3. ¼ cup oil
4. 1 clove garlic, chopped
5. 1 carrot, chopped into ½-inch pieces
6. ½ cup cabbage, chopped
7. 1 cup mushrooms, sliced

8. 1 cup bean sprouts

9. 3 green onions, both parts

Directions

- Incorporate all of the ingredients for the marinade in a resealable bag. Add the chicken pieces and refrigerate for at least 20 minutes. Blend oyster sauce, soy sauce, beef broth and sugar.

- Throw cooked noodles with the sesame oil. Add the ¼ cup of oil to a large skillet or wok and heat over medium-high heat. Add the chicken, reserve the marinade, and cook for about 5 minutes or until cooked through. Remove from the skillet then keep aside.

- Stir extra tablespoon of oil to the skillet if you need to. Cook garlic then add the carrots. Cook for 1 minute. Add the cabbage and mushrooms and cook for about 2 more minutes. Stir the cooked noodles into the pan and cook for another 2 minutes.

- Add the marinade from the resealable bag along with the cooked chicken. Allow to cook for another 3–5 minutes, then serve with rice.

Nutrition: 691 calories 10g fats 34g protein

Tuscan Garlic Chicken

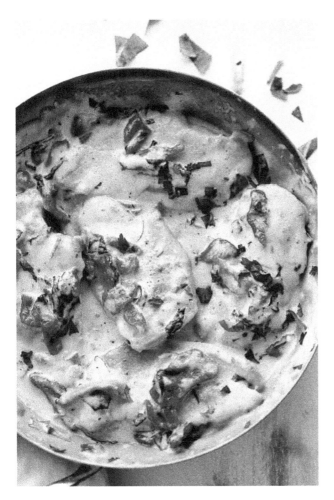

Preparation Time: 15 minutes

Cooking Time: 30 minutes

Servings: 6

Ingredients

Chicken

- 1 cup all-purpose flour

- ½ cup panko bread crumbs
- 1 tablespoon garlic powder
- 2 teaspoons Italian seasoning
- 1 teaspoon sea salt
- 3 boneless skinless chicken breasts
- ½ teaspoon ground black pepper
- ½ teaspoon dried basil
- ½ teaspoon dried oregano
- 2 tablespoons olive oil

Pasta

1. 1-pound fettuccine
2. Sauce
3. 2 tablespoons unsalted butter
4. 4 cloves garlic, minced
5. 1 red bell pepper, cut into 2-inch-long thin strips
6. ½ teaspoon sea salt
7. ¼ teaspoon paprika
8. 1/8 teaspoon ground black pepper
9. 2 tablespoons all-purpose flour
10. 1 cup low-sodium chicken broth
11. 1 cup milk
12. ½ cup half and half
13. 2 cups fresh spinach, roughly chopped

14.   1 cup freshly grated parmesan cheese

Directions

- Preheat oven to 400°F. Line a baking sheet with parchment paper. In a bowl, mix together flour, breadcrumbs, garlic powder, Italian seasoning, salt, pepper, basil, and oregano. Coat the chicken by tossing it in the mixture.

- Cook olive oil in a large skillet over medium heat. Carefully place the chicken in the oil. Sear for 2–3 minutes, making sure not to lose any of the coating. Place chicken onto a baking sheet and then into the oven for 15–20 minutes. While the chicken is baking, cook the fettuccine according to package instructions.

- To make the sauce, cook butter in a large skillet over medium-low heat. Stir in bell pepper and cook for 3–4 minutes. Sprinkle with salt, pepper, and paprika, then add the garlic and sauté for about 1 minute.

- Stir in the flour, then gradually mix the chicken broth, milk and half and half. Bring the heat to medium and simmer. Add the spinach and cook until wilted. Let the sauce thicken and then mix in the parmesan cheese.
- Remove from heat and stir until smooth. Place onto fettuccine and toss together. Slice the chicken and place onto fettuccine. Serve with extra parmesan cheese if desired.

Nutrition: 487 calories 34g protein 7.3g carbohydrates

Stuffed Chicken Marsala

Preparation Time: 25 minutes

Cooking Time: 45 minutes

Servings: 4

Ingredients

Chicken

1. 4 boneless skinless chicken breasts
2. ¾ cup all-purpose flour
3. Salt and pepper to taste
4. ½ cup olive oil
5. Parsley, chopped, for garnish

Stuffing

- ½ cup smoked provolone or gouda cheese, shredded
- ½ pound mozzarella cheese, shredded
- ¼ cup parmesan cheese, grated
- ½ cup breadcrumbs
- 1 teaspoon fresh garlic, minced
- 1 teaspoon red pepper flakes
- 2 tablespoons sun-dried tomatoes, patted dry and roughly chopped
- 3 green onions, thinly sliced

- ¾ cup sour cream

Sauce

1. 1 yellow onion, sliced into strings
2. 1-quart dry marsala wine
3. 1 cup heavy cream
4. ¾ pound button mushrooms, thinly sliced

Directions

- Combine all stuffing ingredients in a bowl. Set aside and preheat oven to 350°F. Make two slices at the thickest part of each chicken breast in order to butterfly it. Flip the chicken over then arrange it flat. Cover with wax paper and pound to about ¼–½ inches in thickness.
- Stuff each chicken breast, but do not overfill. Coat the chicken in salt, pepper, and flour. Cook the chicken in olive oil in a large skillet over medium-high heat. Once cooked, transfer to a baking dish and bake for 15–20 minutes or until the inside is cooked through.

- Using the same large skillet, cook the onions in the chicken drippings for about 2 minutes. Stir in mushrooms and continue to sauté for about 5 more minutes. Deglaze by adding wine to the skillet. Heat the wine until lightly bubbling to reduce it. Continue to cook until the sauce turns brown.
- Heat the heavy cream in the microwave for 20 seconds. Pour it into the pan and heat until it bubbles lightly. Reduce heat to low and simmer for 5 minutes. Remove from heat when the sauce is a rich brown color.
- Serve the sauce over the stuffed chicken and complement the meal with mashed potatoes, if desired. Sprinkle with chopped parsley.

Nutrition: 491 calories 4.6g carbohydrates 31g protein

Chicken Piccata

Preparation Time: 15 minutes

Cooking Time: 15 minutes

Servings: 4 - 6

Ingredients

1. 4 chicken breasts (about 2 pounds)
2. 1 small onion
3. 10 sun-dried tomatoes, cut into strips
4. 1 tablespoon garlic, minced
5. 1½ cups chicken broth
6. Juice of ½ lemon (about 2 tablespoons)
7. ¼ cup capers, rinsed
8. 3 tablespoons butter
9. 1/3 cup heavy cream
10. Salt and pepper to taste
11. ¼ cup olive oil (for frying)

Directions

- Season chicken breasts with salt and pepper. Cook them in a skillet using olive oil over medium-high heat until golden brown and cooked thoroughly (approximately 5–8 minutes on each side). Remove and set aside.

- In the same skillet, sauté the onions, sun-dried tomatoes and garlic until lightly browned. Mix in the chicken broth, lemon juice, and capers. Reduce heat to medium-low and simmer for 10–15 minutes to reduce the sauce.
- Pull away from heat when the sauce has thickened. Add the butter and continue to whisk until melted, then add the cream. Heat for about 30 seconds, then remove. Coat chicken breast in the sauce. Serve.

Nutrition: 501 calories 7.1g carbohydrates 33g protein

Creamy Chicken Breast

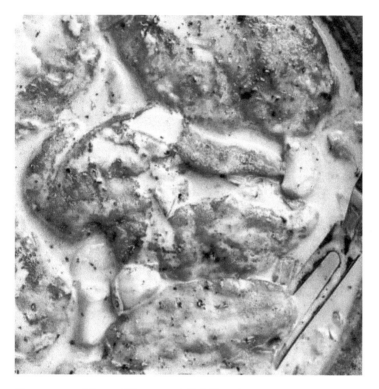

Preparation Time: 10 Minutes

Cooking Time: 20 Minutes

Servings: 4

Ingredients:

1. 1 tablespoon olive oil

2. A pinch of black pepper

3. 2 pounds chicken breasts, skinless, boneless, and cubed

4. 4 garlic cloves, minced

5. 2 and ½ cups low-sodium chicken stock

6. 2 cups coconut cream

7. ½ cup low-fat parmesan, grated

8. 1 tablespoon basil, chopped

Directions:

- Heat-up a pan with the oil over medium-high heat, add chicken cubes, and brown them for 3 minutes on each side.

- Add garlic, black pepper, stock, and cream, toss, cover the pan and cook everything for 10 minutes more.

- Add cheese and basil, toss, divide between plates and serve for lunch. Enjoy!

Nutrition: Calories 221 Fat 6g Fiber 9g Carbs 14g Protein 7g Sodium 197 mg

Indian Chicken Stew

Preparation Time: 60 Minutes

Cooking Time: 20 Minutes

Servings: 4

Ingredients:

1. 1-pound chicken breasts, skinless, boneless, and cubed
2. 1 tablespoon garam masala
3. 1 cup fat-free yogurt
4. 1 tablespoon lemon juice
5. A pinch of black pepper
6. ¼ teaspoon ginger, ground
7. 15 ounces tomato sauce, no-salt-added
8. 5 garlic cloves, minced
9. ½ teaspoon sweet paprika

Directions:

- In a bowl, mix the chicken with garam masala, yogurt, lemon juice, black pepper, ginger, and fridge for 1 hour. Heat-up a pan over medium heat, add chicken mix, toss and cook for 5-6 minutes.

- Add tomato sauce, garlic and paprika, toss, cook for 15 minutes, divide between plates and serve for lunch. Enjoy!

Nutrition: Calories 221 Fat 6g Fiber 9g Carbs 14g Protein 16g Sodium 4 mg

Chicken, Bamboo, and Chestnuts Mix

Preparation Time: 10 Minutes

Cooking Time: 20 Minutes

Servings: 4

Ingredients:

1. 1-pound chicken thighs, boneless, skinless, and cut into medium chunks
2. 1 cup low-sodium chicken stock
3. 1 tablespoon olive oil
4. 2 tablespoons coconut aminos
5. 1-inch ginger, grated
6. 1 carrot, sliced
7. 2 garlic cloves, minced
8. 8 ounces canned bamboo shoots, no-salt-added and drained
9. 8 ounces water chestnuts

Directions:

- Heat-up a pan with the oil over medium-high heat, add chicken, stir, and brown for 4 minutes on each side.

- Add the stock, aminos, ginger, carrot, garlic, bamboo, and chestnuts, toss, cover the pan, and cook everything over medium heat for 12 minutes.
- Divide everything between plates and serve. Enjoy!

Nutrition: Calories 281 Fat 7g Fiber 9g Carbs 14g Protein 14g Sodium 125mg

SEAFOOD RECIPES

Cold Crab Mix

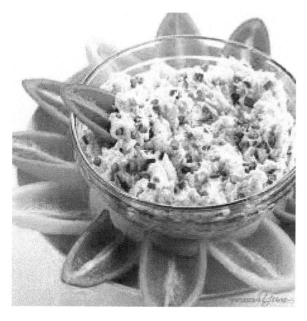

Preparation Time: 5 Minutes

Cooking Time: 15 Minutes

Servings: 4

Ingredients:

1. 2 cups tomatoes, chopped
2. 3 cups watermelon, chopped

3. 3 tbsps. apple cider vinegar

4. 1 tbsp sesame seeds

5. 1 tbsp avocado oil

6. 1 cup crab meat, chopped

Directions:

- Mix all the ingredients together in an enormous bowl and shake well.
- Chill the food for 10 minutes in the refrigerator.

Nutrition: Kcal 111, Sodium 364 mg, Protein 5 g, Carbs 19.5 g, Fat 2 g

Crispy Tilapia with Mediterranean Vegetables

Preparation Time: 5 Minutes

Cooking Time: 35 Minutes

Servings: 4

Ingredients:

1. 1 tbsp olive oil, plus more in a pump sprayer

2. 1 medium yellow onion, chopped

3. 2 cloves garlic, minced

4. 1 normal size zucchini, cut in half lengthwise and then into ½-inch-thick slices

5. 1 medium yellow squash, cut in half lengthwise and then into ½-inch-thick slices

6. 4 plum tomatoes, seeded and cut into ½-inch dice

7. Freshly grated zest of 1 lemon

8. 2 tbsps. fresh lemon juice

9. 1 tbsp chopped fresh oregano, or

10.   1 tsp dried oregano ¼ tsp crushed hot red pepper

11.   4 (5-ounce) tilapia fillets

12.   3 tbsps. panko (Japanese-style bread crumbs), preferably whole-wheat panko

Directions:

- Heat up the oven to 350°F.
- Heat 1 tbsp of oil in a nonstick ovenproof skillet over medium heat.
- Add onion and garlic and cook, occasionally stirring, until just tender, about 3 minutes.
- Add the zucchini and yellow squash and cook until tender, about 3 minutes. Add the tomatoes, lemon zest and juice, oregano and chilly.
- Remove from the heat. Arrange the tilapia fillets on the vegetables.
- Sprinkle with panko and drizzle with oil.
- Cook until tilapia is opaque when flattened in the thickest part with the tip of a knife, about 12 minutes.
- Serve hot.

Nutrition: Kcal 240, Sodium 96 mg, Protein 32 g, Carbs 16 g, Fat 1 g

Crusted Salmon with Horseradish

Preparation Time: 5 Minutes

Cooking Time: 23 Minutes

Servings: 2

Ingredients:

1. 8 ounces salmon fillet
2. 1 ounce's horseradish, grated
3. ¼ tsp ground coriander
4. 1 tsp coconut flakes
5. 1 tbsp olive oil

Directions:

- Combine horseradish, ground cilantro and coconut flakes.
- Then cut the salmon fillet into 2 portions. Heat the olive oil in the pan.
- Put the salmon fillets in the pan and garnish with the horseradish mixture.
- Cook the fish for 5 minutes over medium heat.
- Then turn it over and cook for another 8 minutes.
- Serve right away.

Nutrition: Kcal 220, Sodium 95 mg, Protein 22 g, Carbs 1.5 g, Fat 0.5 g

Cucumber and Seafood Bowl

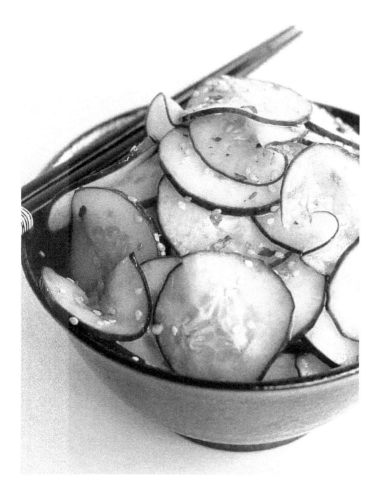

Preparation Time: 5 Minutes

Cooking Time: 25 Minutes

Servings: 3

Ingredients:

1. 2 cucumbers, chopped

2. 1 tsp mustard

3. ½ tsp ground coriander

4. 1 tsp margarine

5. 6 ounces shrimps, peeled

6. 4 ounces salmon, chopped

7. 1 tbsp low-fat yogurt

Directions:

- Heat the margarine in the pan.

- Add the chopped salmon and cook for 2 minutes per side.

- Then add the shrimp and sprinkle the seafood with ground coriander. Close the lid and cook the ingredients for 10 minutes over low heat.

- Then transfer them to serving bowls.

- Add the cucumbers. Mix the yogurt and mustard.

- Sprinkle the food with the mustard mixture and serve.

Nutrition: Kcal 168, Sodium 178 mg, Protein 22 g, Carbs 9.5 g, Fat 5 g

Curry Snapper

Preparation Time: 5 Minutes

Cooking Time: 25 Minutes

Servings: 4

Ingredients:

1. 1-pound snapper fillet, chopped
2. 1 tsp curry powder
3. 1 cup celery stalk, chopped
4. ½ cup low-fat yogurt
5. ¼ cup of water
6. 1 tbsp olive oil

Directions:

- Grill the snapper fillet in olive oil for 2 minutes on each side.
- Then add the celery stalk, curry powder, low-fat yogurt and water.
- Stir the fish until you get a smooth consistency.
- Close the lid and simmer the fish for 10 minutes over medium heat.
- Serve immediately.

Nutrition: Kcal 195, Sodium 105 mg, Protein 29.5 g, Carbs 3 g, Fat 6 g

Dill Steamed Salmon

Preparation Time: 5 Minutes

Cooking Time: 10 Minutes

Servings: 4

Ingredients:

1. 2 tbsps. dill, chopped
2. 1 tbsp low-fat cream cheese
3. 1 tsp chili flakes
4. 1-pound steamed salmon, chopped
5. 1 red onion, diced

Directions:

- Mix up all ingredients in the bowl and carefully stir until homogenous.

Nutrition: Kcal 174, Sodium 62 mg, Protein 23 g, Carbs 3.5 g, Fat 8 g

Fish Salsa

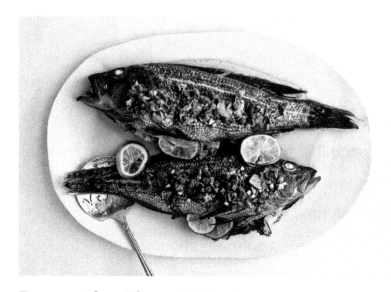

Preparation Time: 5 Minutes

Cooking Time: 10 Minutes

Servings: 12

Ingredients:

1. 1 cup tomatoes, chopped
2. 1-pound salmon, cooked, chopped
3. ½ cup tomatillos, chopped
4. 1 cup watermelon, seedless and chopped
5. ½ cup red onion, chopped
6. 1 cup mango, chopped
7. ¼ cup cilantro, chopped
8. 3 tbsps. lemon juice
9. 2 tbsps. avocado oil

Directions:

- Put all the ingredients in the bowl. Mix the salsa well and let it cool for at least 5 minutes.

Nutrition: Kcal 67, Sodium 17.5 mg, Protein 7 g, Carbs 4 g, Fat 2.5 g

Fish Spread

Preparation Time: 5 Minutes

Cooking Time: 10 Minutes

Servings: 8

Ingredients:

1. 2-pounds trout, boiled
2. 2 tbsps. low-fat cream cheese
3. 1 tbsp fresh dill, chopped
4. 1 tsp minced garlic
5. ¼ cup low-fat yogurt

Directions:

- Put all the ingredients together in the food processor and mix until smooth.
- Transfer the fish spread to the bowl and flatten well.
- Refrigerate the spread for 5 to 10 minutes before serving.

Nutrition: Kcal 231, Sodium 90 mg, Protein 31 g, Carbs 1 g, Fat 10.5 g

Five-Spices Sole

Preparation Time: 5 Minutes

Cooking Time: 22 Minutes

Servings: 8

Ingredients:

1. 3 sole fillets
2. 1 tbsp five-spice seasonings
3. 1 tbsp coconut oil

Directions:

- Rub the sole fillets with the seasonings.
- Then heat up the coconut oil in the pan for 2 minutes.
- Put the sole fillets in the boiling oil and cook for 4.5 minutes on each side.

Nutrition: Kcal 204, Sodium 133 mg, Protein 32 g, Carbs 1 g, Fat 6.5 g

Greek-Styled Salmon

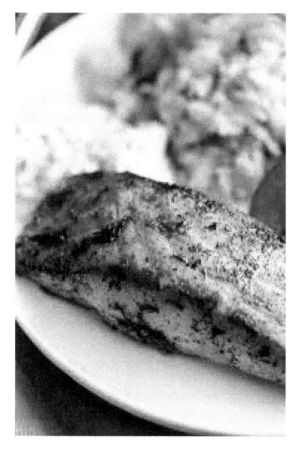

Preparation Time: 5 Minutes

Cooking Time: 20 Minutes

Servings: 4

Ingredients:

1. 4 medium salmon fillets, skinless and boneless

2. 1 tbsp lemon juice

3. 1 tbsp dried oregano

4. 1 tsp dried thyme

5. ¼ tsp onion powder

6. 1 tbsp olive oil

Directions:

- Heat the olive oil in the pan.

- Sprinkle the salmon with dried oregano, thyme, onion powder and lemon juice.

- Spot the fish in the pan and cook on each side for 4 minutes.

Nutrition: Kcal 271, Sodium 80 mg, Protein 34.5 g, Carbs 1 g, Fat 14.5 g

VEGAN RECIPES

Applebee Vegetable Medley

Preparation Time: 15 Minutes

Cooking Time: 10 Minutes

Servings: 4

Ingredients:

1. ½ pound of cold, fresh zucchini, sliced in half moons
2. ½ pound of cold, fresh yellow squash, sliced in half moons
3. ¼ pound of cold red pepper, julienned in strips ¼-inch thick
4. ¼ pound of cold carrots, cut in ¼-inch strips a few inches long
5. ¼ pound of cold red onions, thinly sliced
6. 1 cold, small corn cob, cut crosswise in 1" segments
7. 3 tablespoons of cold butter or margarine
8. 1 teaspoon of salt

9. 1 teaspoon of sugar

10.   ½ teaspoon of granulated garlic

11.   1 teaspoon of Worcestershire sauce

12.   1 teaspoon of soy sauce

13.   2 teaspoons of fresh or dried parsley

Directions:

- Wash, peel, and cut your vegetables as appropriate.
- In a saucepan, heat the butter over medium-high heat.
- Once it is hot, add it the salt, sugar, and garlic.
- Add the carrots, squash, and zucchini, and when they start to soften add the rest of the vegetables and cook for a couple of minutes.
- Add the Worcestershire sauce, soy sauce and parsley.
- Stir to combine and coat the vegetables.
- When all the vegetables are cooked to your preference, serve.

Nutrition: Calories: 170; Fat: 2g; Carbs: 18g; Protein: 15g

PF Chang's Shanghai Cucumbers

Preparation Time: 5 Minutes

Cooking Time: 0 Minutes

Servings: 4

Ingredients:

1. 2 English cucumbers, peeled and chopped
2. 3 tablespoons of soy sauce
3. ½ teaspoon of sesame oil
4. 1 teaspoon of white vinegar
5. Sprinkle of toasted sesame seeds

Directions:

- Stir the soy sauce, sesame oil and vinegar in a serving dish.
- Add the cucumbers and toss to coat.
- Sprinkle with the sesame seeds.

Nutrition: Calories: 70; Fat: 3g; Carbs: 7g; Protein: 4g

Chili Black Bean

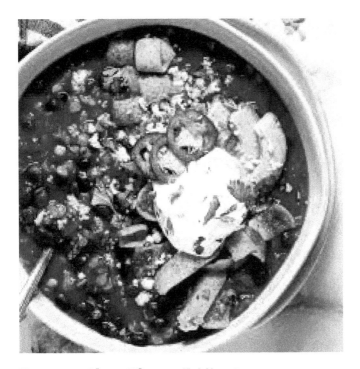

Preparation Time: 5 Minutes

Cooking Time: 25 Minutes

Servings: 6

Ingredients:

1. 2 cans (15.5 ounces each) of black beans
2. ½ teaspoon of sugar
3. 1 teaspoon of ground cumin
4. 1 teaspoon of chili powder
5. ½ teaspoon of garlic powder
6. 2 tablespoons of red onion, diced finely

7. ½ teaspoon of fresh cilantro, minced (optional)

8. ½ cup of water

9. Salt and black pepper to taste

10. Pico de Gallo and or sour cream for garnish (optional)

Directions:

- Combine the beans, sugar, cumin, chili powder, garlic, onion, cilantro (if using), and water in a saucepan and mix well.

- Over medium-low heat, let the bean mixture simmer for about 20-25 minutes. Season with salt and pepper to taste.

- Remove the beans from heat and transfer to serving bowls.

- Garnish with Pico de Gallo and a dollop of sour cream, if desired.

Nutrition: Calories: 143.8; Fat: 0.7g; Carbs: 25.9g; Protein: 9.5.2g

In "N" Out Animal Style Fries

Preparation Time: 10 Minutes

Cooking Time: 30 Minutes

Servings: 6 to 8

Ingredients:

1. 32 ounces of frozen French fries
2. 2 cups of cheddar cheese, shredded
3. 1 large onion, diced
4. 2 tablespoons of raw sugar
5. 2 tablespoons of olive oil
6. 1 ½ cups of mayonnaise
7. ¾ cup of ketchup
8. ¼ cup of sweet relish
9. 1 ½ teaspoons of white sugar
10.   1 ½ teaspoons of apple cider vinegar
11.   ½ teaspoon of salt
12.   ½ teaspoon of black pepper

Directions:

- Preheat oven to 350°F
- Place the oven grill in the middle position.
- Place fries on a large baking sheet and bake in the oven according to package's directions.

- In the time being, warm the olive oil in a large non-stick skillet over medium heat.
- Add the onions and sauté for about 2 minutes until fragrant and soft.
- Add raw sugar and continue cooking until the onions caramelize.
- Remove from heat and set aside.
- Add the mayonnaise, ketchup, relish, white sugar, salt, and black pepper to a bowl and mix until well combined. Set aside.
- Once the fries are cooked, remove from heat and set the oven to broil.
- Sprinkle with the cheddar cheese over the fries and place under the broiler until the cheese melts, about 2–3 minutes.
- Add the cheese fries to serving bowls or plates.
- Add some caramelized onions on top and smother with mayonnaise sauce.
- Serve immediately.

Nutrition: Calories: 750; Fat: 42g; Carbs: 54g; Protein: 19g

KFC Coleslaw

Preparation Time: 15 Minutes

Cooking Time: 0 Minutes

Servings: 10

Ingredients:

1. 8 cups of cabbage, finely diced
2. ¼ cup of carrot, finely diced
3. 2 tablespoons of onions, minced
4. 1/3 cup of granulated sugar
5. ½ teaspoon of salt
6. 1/8 teaspoon of pepper
7. ¼ cup of milk
8. ½ cup of mayonnaise
9. ¼ cup of buttermilk
10.   1½ tablespoons of white vinegar
11.   2½ tablespoons of lemon juice

Directions:

- Mix the carrot, cabbage, and onions in a bowl.
- Place the rest of the ingredients in a blender or food processor and blend until smooth.
- Pour the sauce over the cabbage mixture.

- Place in the fridge for more than a few hours before serving.

Nutrition: Calories: 170; Fat: 12g; Carbs: 14g; Protein: 4g

Cracker Barrel Baby Carrot

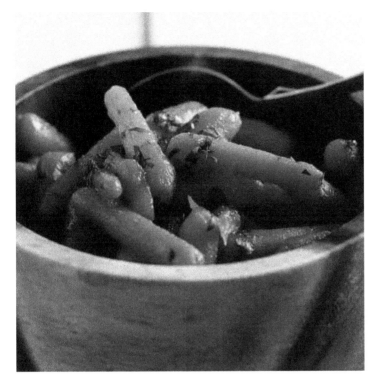

Preparation Time: 5 Minutes

Cooking Time: 45 Minutes

Servings: 6

Ingredients:

1. 1 teaspoon of bacon grease, melted

2. 2 pounds of fresh baby carrots

3. Some water

4. 1 teaspoon of salt

5. ¼ cup of brown sugar

6. ¼ cup of butter, melted

7. ¼ cup of honey

Directions:

1. Heat the bacon grease in a pot.

2. Place the carrots in the grease and sauté for 10 seconds.

3. Cover the carrots with water and add the salt.

4. Bring the whole combination to a boil over medium heat, then reduce the heat to low and let it to simmer for another 30 to 45 minutes.

5. By this time, the carrots should be half cooked.

6. Take away half the water from the pot and add the rest of the ingredients.

7. Keep cooking until the carrots become tender.

8. Transfer to a bowl and serve.

Nutrition: Calories: 80, Fat: 1g, Carbs: 18g, Protein: 1g

Olive Garden Gnocchi with Spicy Tomato

Preparation Time: 10 Minutes

Cooking Time: 40 Minutes

Servings: 4

Ingredients:

Sauce:

- 2 tablespoons of extra virgin olive oil
- 6 fresh garlic cloves
- ½ teaspoon of chili flakes
- 1 cup of dry white wine
- 1 cup of chicken broth
- 2 cans (14.5 ounces each) of tomatoes
- ¼ cup of fresh basil, chopped
- ¼ cup of sweet creamy butter, cut into 1-inch cubes, chilled
- ½ cup of parmesan cheese, freshly grated

Pasta:

- 1 pound of gnocchi
- Salt, to taste
- Black pepper, freshly crushed, to taste

Directions:

1. Place the garlic, olive oil, and chili flakes in a cold pan and cook over medium heat.

2. Once the garlic starts turning golden brown, add the wine and broth and bring the mixture to a simmer.

3. After about 10 minutes, the broth should be halved.

4. When that happens, add in the tomatoes and basil and then let the sauce continue simmering for another 30 minutes.

5. When the sauce has condensed, set it aside to cool for 3 minutes.

6. After 3 minutes, place the sauce in a blender, and add the butter and parmesan.

7. Purée everything together and set aside.

8. Prepare the pasta by boiling the gnocchi in a large pot.

9. When it is cooked, strain the pasta and mix with the sauce.

10. Transfer everything to a plate and serve.

Nutrition: Calories: 285.8; Fat: 18.9g; Carbs: 12.1g; Protein: 8.4g; Sodium: 476.9mg

Chipotle Sofritas

Preparation Time: 10 Minutes

Cooking Time: 25 Minutes

Servings: 4

Ingredients:

Mexican Spice Mix:

- ½ teaspoon of dried oregano leaves
- 2 teaspoons of ancho chili powder, ground
- 1 teaspoon of cumin, ground
- ½ teaspoon of coriander, ground
- ½ teaspoon of kosher salt

Sofritas:

- 1 tablespoon of avocado or olive oil
- ½ medium onion, diced
- 2 garlic cloves, minced
- 1 teaspoon of chipotle chili in adobo sauce, minced
- 1 tablespoon of mild Hatch chili, diced
- 1 tablespoon of Mexican Spice Mix
- 2 tablespoons of tomato paste
- 1 package (16 ounces) of organic extra firm tofu, drained, dried, crumbled

- 1 cup of your favorite Mexican beer
- Salt and black pepper to taste
- Tortillas and lime wedges for garnish

Directions:

1. Place all the Mexican Spice Mix ingredients in a container or plastic bag and shake to mix.
2. Sauté the onion and garlic in oil over medium heat for 5 minutes.
3. Mix in both the chilies and the spice mix and sauté for another minute.
4. Pour in the tomato paste and cook for a minute.
5. Add the rest of the ingredients and cook for 5 more minutes.
6. Taste and regulate seasoning with salt and pepper if required.
7. Remove the mixture from heat, transfer to a bowl, and then serve with tortillas and thin lime wedges.

Nutrition: Calories: 470, Fat: 19g, Carbs: 59g, Protein: 16g, Sodium: 1160mg

Melting Pot Green Goddess Dip

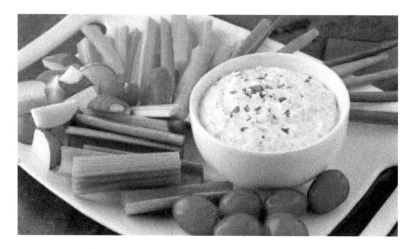

Preparation Time: 5 Minutes

Cooking Time: 5 Minutes

Servings: 12

Ingredients:

- 8 ounces of cheese, sliced
- 1/2 cup of milk
- 1/4 cup of cream
- 2 tbsp. of onion
- 2 tbsp. of parsley
- 2 tbsp. of chives

Directions:

1. Microwave cheese and milk in a healthy container for 2–4 minutes, whisking after each minute, before adding the cream cheese.

2. Melt and mix smoothly.

3. Stir in sour cream, cabbage, chives, and parsley.

4. Refrigerate before serving and enjoy!

Nutrition: Calories: 85, Fat: 7.8g, Carbs: 1.6g, Protein: 1.6g

Applebee Onion Peels

Preparation Time: 5 Minutes

Cooking Time: 25 Minutes

Servings: 4 to 6

Ingredients:

Horseradish dipping sauce:

- 1/2 cup of mayonnaise
- 1 tbsp. of prepared horseradish
- 2 tsp. of white vinegar
- 1 tsp. of water
- 1 tsp. of paprika
- 1 tsp. of ketchup
- 1/4 tsp. of black pepper
- 1/8 tsp. of dried oregano
- 1/8 tsp. of cayenne
- 1/4 tsp. of garlic powder
- 1/4 tsp. of onion powder

Batter:

- 5–6 cups of shortening
- 1 large onion
- 1/2 cup of all-purpose flour
- 1/2 cup of Progresso Plain Bread Crumbs

- 1/2 tsp. of salt
- 1/2 tsp. of black pepper
- 1 1/2 cups of milk

Directions:

1. Make horseradish dipping sauce, mixing ingredients with a whisk in a medium cup.
2. Then blend the sauce until smooth, cover, and chill.
3. Heat the shortening on a deep fryer to 350°F.
4. Slice the end of the stem and the end of the root off the onion, then cut through the onion, slice it in half with the onion lying on a flat side. Slice each half 4 to 5 times more to make onion wedges in a spoken fashion.
5. Separate pieces of an onion.
6. Mix all the dry fixings into a medium bowl to make batter.
7. Whisk in the milk until smooth batter then let the batter sit for 5 minutes. It should grow thicker.
8. Then again whisk the batter.

9. Dip pieces of onion in the batter, when the oil is hot, let some of the batter drip off, and then cautiously drop the piece of coated onion into the hot oil.

10. Repeat for 1 to 2 minutes, or until light brown, frying 8 to 12 at a time.

11. Drain onto a towel rack or notebook.

12. Repeat until the onion is removed, stack the newer lots on top of the old lots to keep them dry.

13. Serve fried onion slices on a plate or in a paper-coated basket with horseradish dipping sauce on the side when they are all done.

Nutrition: Calories: 234, Fat: 14g, Carbs: 22g, Protein: 5g

SAUCE AND DRESSING RECIPES

Abuelo's Jalapeño Cheese Fritters

Preparation Time: 15 minutes

Cooking Time: 20 minutes

Servings: 8

Ingredients

Fritters

- 1 (8-ounce) package cream cheese, softened
- ½ cup Monterrey cheese, shredded
- ½ cup cheddar cheese, shredded
- 3 jalapeños, deseeded and finely chopped
- 1 teaspoon Lawry's seasoning
- Oil for frying

Breading

1. 3 cups breadcrumbs
2. ¼ cup all-purpose flour

3. Egg Wash

4. 2 eggs

5. ¼ cup water

Directions

- Grease and preheat at 300 degrees. Blend all the ingredients then form the mixture into 1-inch balls (makes approximately 20 balls). Place onto the prepared sheet and set aside.

- Beat the eggs and water together until slightly frothy; set aside. To two separate bowls, add the flour and breadcrumbs; set aside.

Assembling

1. Roll the balls in the flour first. Dunk each ball into the egg wash and then into the breadcrumbs. Toss until evenly coated. Cook the oil at 350°F and fry the balls until evenly golden brown. Drain the balls on a paper towel. Serve with your favorite dip.

Nutrition: 636 calories 47g total fats 30g protein

Baja Fresh's Guacamole

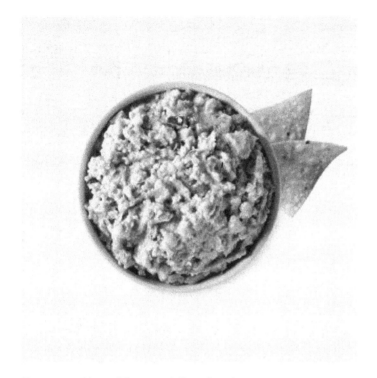

Preparation Time: 10 minutes

Cooking Time: 0 minute

Serving: 4

Ingredients

- Flesh of 3 avocados, chopped
- 2 tablespoons lime juice
- ¾ teaspoon salt
- ½ teaspoon ground cumin
- ¼ teaspoon cayenne powder
- 1 small onion, finely chopped

- 2 Roma tomatoes, seeded and diced
- 1 tablespoon chopped cilantro

Directions

1. In a medium bowl, mash the avocados. Mix in the lime juice and Stir well. Stir in the salt, cumin, cayenne, onion, tomatoes, and cilantro.
2. Allow guacamole sit at room temperature for about 30 minutes for the flavors to blend.

Nutrition: 701 calories 49g total fats 31g protein

Chipotle's Guacamole

Preparation Time: 10 minutes

Cooking Time: 0 minutes

Serving: 6

Ingredients

- 1 medium jalapeño pepper, seeded and deveined, finely chopped
- 1 cup diced red onion
- 2 tablespoons fresh cilantro, chopped finely
- 8 ripe avocados
- 8 teaspoons freshly squeezed lime juice
- 1 teaspoon kosher salt

Directions

1. Chop avocado in half and take out the flesh. Mix in the jalapeño pepper, onion, and cilantro. Drizzle the lime juice. Season it with salt. Pound avocado with the rest of the ingredients until desired consistency is achieved. Seal it with plastic wrap before serving.

Nutrition: 674 calories 37g total fats 26g protein

Chili Con Queso

Preparation Time: 5 minutes

Cooking Time: 5 minutes

Servings: 8

Ingredients

- 1 block Velveeta® cheese
- ½ teaspoon granulated garlic
- 1 (4 ½-ounce) canned diced green chilies, drained
- 1 (4 ½-ounce) can pimiento peppers, drained
- 1 jalapeño pepper, minced
- Nacho chips, for serving

Directions

1. In a microwaveable bowl, melt the Velveeta, checking and stirring often. Stir in the other ingredients. Serve warm with nacho chips.

Nutrition: 637 calories 46g total fats 27g protein

Chipotle's Queso Dip

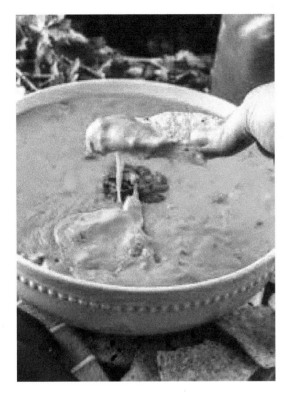

Preparation Time: 15 minutes

Cooking Time: 2 hours

Servings: 8

Ingredients

- 1 cup cheddar, cubed
- 1 cup American cheese, cubed
- 1 cup Monterey Jack, cubed
- 1 cup heavy cream
- 2 poblano peppers

- 1 large Roma tomato, halved
- 1 teaspoon paprika
- 1 teaspoon garlic powder
- ¼ teaspoon cayenne pepper
- ½ teaspoon black pepper
- 1 tablespoon olive oil
- Tortilla chips to serve

Directions

2. Grease the baking dish with oil and preheat at 400 degrees. Place the tomatoes and poblano pepper in the prepared baking dish and bake until the skins are blackened.

3. Although the veggies are in the oven, mix remaining ingredients in a pot and let simmer on low. Once cooked, set aside and let cool at room temperature for about 10 minutes.

4. Remove the skins and transfer to a blender. Blend until pureed. Add the pureed veggies to the cheese mixture; mix well and continue cooking for 2 hours. Serve hot with tortilla chips.

Nutrition: 677 calories 41g total fats 30g protein

Don Pablo's White Chili

Preparation Time: 10 minutes

Cooking Time: 30 minutes

Servings: 4

Ingredients

1. 1 tablespoon olive oil
2. 8 ounces chicken breast
3. 1 small onion
4. 3 cloves garlic
5. 1 red bell pepper
6. 2 (15-ounce) cans white beans
7. 1 (4-ounce) can green chilies
8. ½ teaspoon ground cumin
9. 2 teaspoons chili powder
10. 2 cups chicken broth
11. 2 tablespoons lime juice
12. 2 tablespoons fresh cilantro
13. ½ cup salsa (optional)

Directions

- In a stock pot, warm the oil. Sauté the chicken pieces until they are lightly browned.

- Add the onion and cook to soften. Stir in the garlic and red bell pepper and cook until fragrant.
- Add the beans, green chilies, cumin, chili powder, and broth. Heat up to simmer and cook for 15 minutes. Pour in lime juice and cilantro, and serve garnished with a spoonful of salsa, if desired.

Nutrition: 669 calories 43g total fats 30g protein

Chili's Original Chili

Preparation Time: 15 minutes

Cooking Time: 1 hour 30 minutes

Servings: 4

Ingredients

Spice Blend

1. ½ cup chili powder
2. 1/8 cup salt
3. 1/8 cup ground cumin
4. 1 tablespoon paprika
5. 1 teaspoon ground black pepper
6. 1 teaspoon garlic powder
7. 1 teaspoon of cayenne pepper

Chili

- 4 pounds chuck, ground for chili
- 3¼ cups water
- 16 ounces tomato sauce
- 1½ cups yellow onions, chopped
- 1 tablespoon cooking oil

Masa Harina

1. 1 cup water
2. 1 tablespoon masa harina

3. Sliced green onions for garnish, if desired

Directions

- Put all the spice blend ingredients in a bowl. Mix thoroughly and set the bowl aside. Cook the meat at medium heat in a stock pot until it is brown. While the meat is cooking, thoroughly mix together the spice mix, water, and tomato sauce.

- Stir in spice mixture to the browned meat and bring to a boil. When chili is about to boil, sauté the onions in oil over medium heat for the meantime. When the chili is boiling and the onions are translucent, add the onions to the chili and stir.

- Set heat to low and let the chili to simmer for an hour, stirring the mixture every 15 minutes. In a bowl, mix the masa harina ingredients together. When the chili has been cooking for an hour, add the masa harina mixture to the chili and cook for another 10 minutes.

- Transfer the chili to a bowl, garnish green onions, if desired, and serve.

Nutrition: 681 calories 48g total fats 32g protein

2-Ingredient Tahini Paste

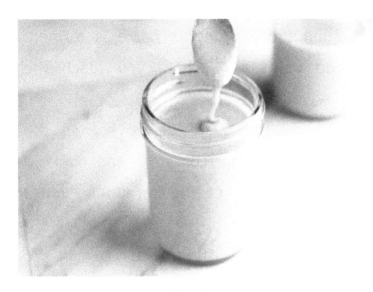

Preparation Time: 15 minutes

Cooking Time: 30 minutes

Servings: 16

Ingredients:

1. 1 cup of hulled sesame seeds
2. 3 tbsps. extra virgin olive oil

Directions:

- Pour the sesame seeds into a pan and roast over medium-high heat, stirring regularly, until the seeds are brown.

- Let seeds to cool then situate them in a blender/food processor. Drizzle in 3 tbsps. of olive oil and process until a paste is formed. Slowly add in more oil until you reach the consistency you'd prefer.
- Thoroughly stir the paste before storing the tahini in an airtight jar/container and place in the refrigerator. Tahini can be stored for about 3 months.

Nutrition: 36 Calories 7g Fat 1g Protein

Spicy Mexican Barbecue Sauce

Preparation Time: 15 minutes

Cooking Time: 15 minutes

Servings: 12

Ingredients:

1. 2/3 olive oil
2. 1 onion, diced
3. ½ tbsp garlic paste
4. 1 ½ tsps. of salt
5. 1 chili pepper, seeded & diced
6. 2 tomatoes, peeled & chopped
7. 2 tbsps. of chili powder
8. 2 tbsps. of sugar
9. ¼ cup of vinegar
10.   ¼ cup of beer

Directions:

- Cook oil in a pan over medium heat. Drop in the onions and fry until browned.
- Stir in the garlic, chili, chili powder, salt and tomatoes. Simmer for 4 minutes

- Pour in the sugar, vinegar and beer and let it simmer for 10 minutes, stirring regularly. Remove from heat and let it cool.

Nutritional: 126 Calories 11.6g Fat 0.7g Protein

Tangy French Remoulade Sauce

Preparation Time: 15 minutes

Cooking Time: 15 minutes

Servings: 8

Ingredients:

1. ¾ cup of mayonnaise
2. 1 ½ tbsp of cornichon or dill relish
3. 1 tsp of finely chopped capers
4. 1 tbsp of lemon juice
5. 1 tbsp of mustard (preferably Dijon)
6. 2 tsp of chopped parsley
7. 1 dash of hot sauce
8. ½ tsp of salt

Direction:

- Incorporate mayonnaise with the cornichon, capers, lemon juice, mustard, salt and parsley together. Stir in the hot sauce and then cover with plastic wrap. Place in the refrigerator until needed.

Nutrition: 146 Calories 1g Carbohydrates 16g Fat

DESSERT RECIPES

Olive Garden® Lemon Cream Cake

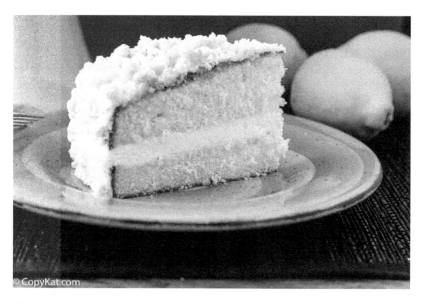

Preparation Time: 10 minutes

Cooking Time: 30 minutes

Servings: 4-5

Ingredients:

Cooking spray

Cake:

1. 1 (16.25 ounce) package white cake mix

2. ¾ cup milk

3. 1 tablespoon milk

4. 2 eggs

5. 3 1/2 tablespoons vegetable oil

Crumb Topping:

6. 2 tablespoons butter, melted

7. 1/2 teaspoon vanilla extract

Filling:

8. 4 ounces cream cheese, softened

9. 2/3Cup confectioners' sugar, divided, plus more for dusting

10.   3 tablespoons lemon juice

11.   1 teaspoon grated lemon zest

12.   2 cups heavy whipping cream

Directions:

- Preheat oven up to 175 degrees C (350 degrees F). Spray the cooking spray on the bottom side of a 10-inch spring form pan.

- Measure 1 mix of cupcake; set aside to top with the crumb. In a large bowl, put the remaining cake mixture; add 3/4 cup plus one tablespoon of milk, eggs, and oil. Using an electric mixer, beat cake mixture until batter is thoroughly mixed, around 2 minutes. Pour batter into the ready-made tub.
- Mix the butter which should be melted and vanilla extract in a bowl; whisk in 1 cupcake mixture until mixture is crumbly. Sprinkle the crumbs with the cake batter on top.
- Bake in the preheated oven until crisp, 30 to 35 minutes, a toothpick inserted in the center of the cake comes out. Heat cake in the pan until room temperature.
- In a bowl, mix cream cheese, 1/3 cup sugar, lemon juice, and lemon zest until smooth and creamy. Beat the cream and the remaining 1/3 cup sugar in a separate bowl using an electric mixer until stiff peaks form. Turn mixture of cream cheese into whipped cream.

- Take the cake off the spring form plate. Use a serrated knife, cut the cake horizontally into two layers, and remove the top layer. Place the filling onto the bottom sheet of the cake; place the top cake overfilling. Cool the cake down for at least 4 hours. Until serving, sprinkle the cake with more confectioners' sugar.

Nutrition: Calories 676; Carbs 89g; Protein 8g; Fat 32g

Nothing Bundt Cakes® White Chocolate Raspberry

Preparation Time: 20 minutes

Cooking Time: 10 minutes

Servings: 5-6

Ingredients:

1. Chopped into small cubes, 200g butter, plus extra for greasing
2. 100g white chocolate, broken into pieces
3. Four large eggs
4. 200g caster sugar
5. 200g self-rising flour
6. 175g raspberries, fresh or frozen

For the ganache:

7. 200g white chocolate, chopped
8. 250ml double cream
9. A little icing sugar, for dusting

Directions:

- Heat oven to fan/gas 4, 180C/160C. Grease and line the 2 x 20 cm round base with loose-bottomed cake tins. In a heat-proof mixing bowl, place the butter and chocolate, set over a pan of barely simmering water, and allow to melt gradually, stirring occasionally.

- Once butter and chocolate have melted, remove from heat and cool for 1-2 minutes, then beat with an electric whisk in the eggs and sugar. Fold and raspberries in the starch.

- Pour the mixture gently into the tins and bake for 20-25 minutes or until golden brown and a skewer inserted in the center is clean (Don't be fooled by their juiciness, the raspberries the leave a residue on the skewer). Pullout the cakes from the oven & allow for 10 minutes of cooling in the tins before placing on a wire rack.

- To make the ganache, place the chocolate over a pan of barely simmering water in a heatproof bowl with 100ml of the cream on top. Remove until the chocolate has melted into the sugar, and leave a smooth, shiny ganache on you. You need to leave the ganache at room temperature to cool, then beat in the rest of the cream.
- Sandwich them together with the chocolate ganache after the cakes have cooled. Just before serving, sprinkle them with icing sugar.

Nutrition: Calories 410; Fat 40g; Carbs 68g; Protein 3g

Longhorn Steakhouse® Chocolate Mousse Cake

Preparation Time: 10 minutes

Cooking Time: 25 minutes

Servings: 6-7

Ingredients:

1. 1 (18.25 ounce) chocolate cake mix pack
2. 1 (14 ounces) can sweeten condensed milk
3. 2 (1 ounce) squares unsweetened chocolate, melted
4. 1/2 cup of cold water
5. 1 (3.9 ounces) package instant chocolate pudding mix
6. 1 cup heavy cream, whipped

Directions:

- Preheat oven up to 175 degrees C (350 degrees F). Prepare and bake cake mix on two 9-inch layers according to package directions. Cool off and pan clean.

- Mix the sweetened condensed milk and melted chocolate together in a big tub. Stir in water slowly, then pudding instantly until smooth. Chill in for 30 minutes, at least.
- Remove from the fridge the chocolate mixture, and whisk to loosen. Fold in the whipped cream and head back to the refrigerator for at least another hour.
- Place one of the cake layer onto a serving platter. Top the mousse with 1 1/2 cups, then cover with the remaining cake layer. Frost with remaining mousse, and cool until served. Garnish with chocolate shavings or fresh fruit.

Nutrition: Calories 530; Fat 57g; Carbs 5g; Protein 12g

The Cheesecake Factory® Pumpkin Cheesecake

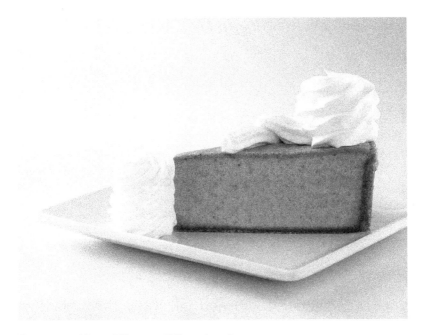

Preparation Time: 30 minutes

Cooking Time: 40 minutes

Servings: 6-7

Ingredients:

1. 2 (8 ounce) packages cream cheese, softened
2. 1/2 cup white sugar
3. 1/2 teaspoon vanilla extract
4. Two eggs
5. 1 (9 inches) prepared graham cracker crust
6. 1/2 cup pumpkin puree

7. 1/2 teaspoon ground cinnamon

8. One pinch ground clove

9. One pinch ground nutmeg

10.   1/2 cup frozen whipped topping, thawed

Directions:

- Preheat the oven up to 325 ° F (165 ° C).

- The vanilla, cream cheese & the sugar are mixed in a big tub. Beat to smooth. Blend one at a time into shells. Remove 1 cup of batter and spread to the crust bottom; set aside.

- Add the remaining mixture with the pumpkin, cinnamon, cloves, and nutmeg, and stir gently until well blended. Spread carefully through the crust over the batter.

- Bake 35 to 40 minutes in the already preheated oven, or until the center is nearly set. Enable to cool, then refrigerate overnight or for 3 hours. Until serving cover with whipped topping.

Nutrition: Calories 1050; Fat 78g; Carbs 76g; Protein 11g

Famous Dave® Cornbread Muffins

Preparation Time: 10 minutes

Cooking Time: 25 minutes

Servings: 6-7

Ingredients:

1. 1/2 cup butter softened
2. 2/3Cup white sugar
3. 1/4 cup honey
4. Two eggs
5. 1/2 teaspoon salt
6. 1 1/2 cups all-purpose flour
7. ¾ cup cornmeal
8. 1/2 teaspoon baking powder
9. 1/2 cup milk
10.   ¾ cup frozen corn kernels, thawed

Directions:

- Preheat oven to 400 grades F (200 grades C). Grease or 12 cups of muffins on deck.

- Cream the butter, sugar, honey, eggs, and salt together in a big pot. Add in rice, cornmeal, and baking powder, blend well. Stir in corn and milk. Pour the yield into prepared muffin cups or spoon them.
- Bake for 20 to 25 minutes in a preheated oven until a toothpick inserted in the center of a muffin comes out clean.

Nutrition: Calories 270; Fat 37g; Carbs 12g; Protein 4g

CONCLUSION

Thank you for you had finished this book.

Copycat Recipes are recipes that are copied from restaurants, prepared by home cooks, but sold to the public as the actual restaurant's recipe.

In this book, I have enlightened how you can make these recipes (of course, there are some exceptions.) This book doesn't contain any comments on those recipes about whether they tasted good or gross. Everybody has different tastes, so it should be up to you to decide whether they look would be tasty or if they're disgusting! There are many types of cuisine, and what one person hates another might love it. So, try these foods yourself and decide what you think about them ~ It's time for your taste buds to wake up!

Here are tips that I want to give you with regards to cooking copycat recipes:

- Learn the rule of combining things. Such as, "Cook soup in a lot of water" or "Add meat to the rice."

- Cook slowly. Add spices or seasonings to the foods after you've melted them in a small saucepan and then you have an idea how much more they need to cook, but it cannot be cooked until it smells right, otherwise it will taste gross.

- Don't add eggs unless they're cooking for a long time (such as making omelet.)

- Learn that certain ingredients are not good together. For example, onion and carrots are terrible when cooked together because the onion will take away all the flavor from carrots and onions together should be cooked separately ~ The explanation is really simple! There's a term called synergy which means that foods do not work well together because it causes discoloration such as "green color."

- Use less salt or sugar if so desired (some people say that they can't eat sweet food without looking up sugar content on their phone because they will feel high from eating too much sugar.)

- Do not mix the flavors together (such as curry and soy sauce.)

- Separate your foods by their ingredients (such as meat and vegetables) into different pots. This prevents everything from become mushy! 8.

- Add lemon juice to food that's about to burn.

- How to make bread or just flat bread or tacos (corn tortilla): Add the ingredients in the order of liquid, then flour, then spices and baking powder.

- If you want to make mashed potatoes, add milk or cream before cooking them ~ I don't know why, but they say that it makes mashed potatoes taste better!

- Some foods cannot be prepared without oil such as French fries, ravioli and onion rings--I read a lot of stories about this online so it is true!

- How to easily differentiate between meats such as chicken breast and chicken thighs: The skin of chicken thighs is darker than chicken breast meat

- The easiest way to get cleared of grease in food is putting paper towel on a plate with other food on top of it!

I hope you had enjoyed all of the recipes included in this book.

Thank you.

CPSIA information can be obtained
at www.ICGtesting.com
Printed in the USA
BVHW050551120421
604724BV00002B/178